CONTENTS

THE PD BACKGROUND	3
WHAT ABOUT A CURE?	6
HOW IS PD FIRST NOTICED?	7
WHAT BRINGS PD OUT INTO THE OPEN?	9
SOME OUTWARDS SIGNS OF PD	10
BODY LANGUAGE	12
ON/OFF AND ITS PROBLEMS	17
SOME PD PROBLEMS	19
DEPRESSION	19
HALLUCINATION	20
SWALLOWING	20
SPEECH AND SPEECH THERAPY	21
SUPPORTING SERVICES	23
TREATMENT OF SUFFERERS FROM PARKINSON'S DISEASE	25
A FEW MISUNDERSTANDINGS	27
DO OUTSIDERS REALLY UNDERSTAND PD AND TREAT THE SUFFERER AND CARER WITH KINDNESS?	28
THOUGHTLESS OR UNINTENTIONAL KINDNESSES	29
THE HOME CARER, OR INSIDER - HOW YOU CAN HELP THEM	30
GETTING OUT AND ABOUT	32
FOR THE CARER, SOME THINGS THAT MAY HELP	34
IF YOU REALLY WANT TO HELP A PARKINSONIAN FAMILY ...	37
WORDS THAT CAN CONFUSE THE LAYMAN	40
THANK YOU AND GOODBYE	41
JIM	42
A MESSAGE FROM A SUFFERER	43

At the back are a few items of interest
including a Personal Passport sheet about the sufferer.
If this was completed and kept up to date
it might be of great value if the sufferer and carer
had to be parted for any reason.

PLEASE
READ NOTES OVERLEAF BEFORE OPENING THIS BOOKLET

PLEASE NOTE

This booklet is written to help Parkinsonian families by explaining to people who may be employed in caring for them what it is like when PD takes over a family.

It is not bedtime reading and should not be handed to a sufferer or carer unless you are absolutely certain that it will help them. But please do pass it round among your friends who also work to help people with PD. It is no good left on a shelf.

PD attacks male and female equally but we cannot write "he" or "she" each time a personal pronoun has to be used. I have come across a charming phrase in a St John paper which says that 'for the purpose of the text the male term shall embrace the female'. Please accept that throughout this text the male term will be embracing the female (and the female the male for the matter of that) in the same way.

PD people, I know, deserve a better write up than I have been able to give them herein and I would like to apologise for any untoward statement I may have made and to express my deep admiration for the way in which they cope with so many tedious daily chores.

If this booklet in any way eases their problems it will have been worth every drop of midnight oil which has been burnt in writing it.

Pam McClintock

THE PD BACKGROUND
(and a look at the future)

Dr Parkinson, a London doctor, learned about PD by observing its effect on people. Finally he wrote a thesis on it in 1818. Because he was the first person to identify it as an independent condition it became known as Dr Parkinson's Disease. The 'Dr' was dropped a long time ago, and I think we would all like to drop the 'Disease'. In fact most of us now do drop it, calling it simply 'Parkinson's' or 'PD'.

With no training in PD or qualification of any sort I, too, have learnt all I know trying to help people with PD and, of course, their families. They have taught me all I know. PD is rather a lonely condition, people may become housebound and, because it is such a bizarre condition, everyone's PD causes different problems. It is therefore almost impossible to compare notes with fellow sufferers. Because I have visited so many - over four hundred - in the last ten years I believe that I have gained some insight into the condition which could be of value to other PD families.

Although you may feel that it is arrogant of me, an amateur, to think that I may have a greater understanding than the professionals, I feel that I should not withhold anything that I may have learnt that could possibly help others to improve their quality of life The people that I try to help at present live in such a large area that I use four different telephone codes and spend quite a bit of time in my car. Some sufferers live in towns, many live down unmade roads, sometimes I find three or four bunched together in close proximity, other times I have to drive quite a distance to visit one family. Most are living at home, a few in Residential Care and one or two in Nursing Homes.

I have the deepest admiration for almost all sufferers and their families and wish I could do more for them. Hence this booklet.

PD is really a condition, for which at present there is no cure, although there are many ways of alleviating the distress and even delaying its progress. Like other modern treatments the medication can sometimes have tiresome side effects. All PD medication is the result of comparatively recent research, and the curtain is only gradually being drawn aside, but one day, perhaps in your lifetime if not in mine ...

PD has been around for a long time. It is mentioned in the Bible, in Matthew, Mark, Luke and the Acts as the 'palsy'. In the 1820's soon after Dr Parkinson wrote his thesis, an ancestor of mine, a parson and the heir to his brother's estate, developed it. He became what his rather possessive twin sister called 'sadly nervous'. She said he could no longer 'carve his food' and would not eat with strangers. He 'shut himself away' but this was actually because his housekeeper took control of his house, refusing admission to relatives and after his death she produced a Will that left everything to the man her daughter was going to marry! Luckily this Will was proved to be a forgery after some years of litigation.

I have looked at his handwriting in the Parish Registers way back in the 1820's, and there is little doubt in my mind that it deteriorated over the years, just as PD handwriting does today. He was very much a family man and I do not think that the housekeeper would have been able to rule his house, and shut the door on his relatives if he had not been 'sadly nervous' with PD, for in his obituary notices he is described as an independent magistrate who always made up his mind for himself. I am afraid that there is not room here to tell how the wicked housekeeper's family forged the Will.

Just after the First World War an especially vicious influenza swept through England. It is said to have killed more people than died in the trenches. This influenza could have been one of the causes of a certain type of PD which often lies dormant until the person passes middle age. Certainly many people who were young in 1919 are not suffering from PD.

As an amateur historian it interests me to check on the 'flu epidemics and then look to see what effect this had decades later.

Several people that I know think that their PD developed after they had suffered a 'flu-like illness in the Far East. They are now mostly in their 50's and 60's.

Sometimes, if PD starts with a hand tremor and the person goes on to have an unsteady gait, people may think they have taken to the bottle. I knew a Brigadier with an excellent war record, and a very nice person too, who became like that shortly after his wife died, and I must say we were all rather distressed and wondered about him.

In 1954/55, I think, Asian flu swept around the world. It was very infectious and it was easily spread, especially as air travel had become the norm and people carried the infection with them when they flew from A to B. In Nigeria it suddenly hit Kano (a big staging post on the African routes) when someone flew in who was already hatching the flu. People went down like ninepins and in the large African city it was known as 'the stranger who entered every gate'. The markets and the busy streets became silent and deserted, and sheep and goats browsed where the lorries and cars would otherwise have surely killed them. (At least I am told it was like this; I did not see it myself because I, too, had been struck down!)

I wonder whether, in years to come, those of us who had Asian flu will develop Parkinson's. We will have to wait and see.

What really does cause PD? Are there many causes, or is there one cause that is so obvious that we have not yet thought of it? Is it environment, background, trauma? Has it lain dormant in our bodies for years and been suddenly triggered into action, or is it caught from others, or ...?

I do not know; does anybody? But I do know that before PD becomes obvious to others, or even to the sufferers themselves, 80% of the cells of a certain part of the brain may have been destroyed and brain cells cannot be replaced.

If the PD has developed slowly, so slowly that no-one has noticed, as many cases do, that will mean that the <u>cause</u> could well be lost and forgotten, for as we grow older and our lifestyle changes, we forget our way of life when we were young. And the modern researcher may well not have been alive then, and would find it hard even to understand our pre-war way of life, much of which is commonplace to us oldies.

If an older person has just been diagnosed as having PD it may be difficult for him to answer questions about his childhood or about his time in the Services or as an evacuee. In fact the researchers may not be able to ask the right question because things have changed so much. They would find it difficult to understand pre-World War Two and people have moved about so much since then that 'roots' are often difficult to trace. Progress has changed our lives out of all recognition and I think it is not at all surprising that old people suffer from dementia; they have had to adjust to so much in their lifetime.

And do modern researchers know enough about the common way of life in the good old days? Do they know about Iodine Lockets, which we all wore, or the soft leadlike toothpaste tubes? Do they remember about the dangers of tinned meat from South America or the cheap tin saucepans that could be got for 6d, or the anthracite stoves in Servicemen's huts during the war?

I remember them especially because when I was in the Forces some portable anthracite stoves were used to try and prevent the water in our Ablution Huts from freezing and once I was nearly overcome by the fumes. Will I develop PD? And would I have remembered about this if a researcher has asked me? It was only by chance that I found a letter about it recently.

In one of Agatha Christie's books the plot hangs on an 'open secret' - a secret that everybody knew and thought everyone else knew, so that they never mentioned it to M Poirot. Perhaps the secret of PD is like that: we all did or knew something that is so ordinary that we think everyone else knows it.

An unusual number of people who have been to the Far East seem to have developed PD. I know of three ex-servicemen who have been awarded a pension because it is believed that their PD was caused by their Far Eastern service - but not, surprisingly enough, a sufferer who spent some years in a Japanese Prisoner of War camp.

Again, during the war when matches were not available, many people used a petrol cigarette lighter. In drawing in the flame to light the cigarette they must also have drawn in the petrol fumes. Could this have started the PD?

These are only thoughts, which are mentioned here to start you off thinking and listening to PD families. One thing I do know for certain - almost every family afflicted by PD are very nice people indeed. This is not a layabout's disease. PD people are the sort of people who have worked hard all their lives, self-disciplined and caring - and they are often very good gardeners too. Many have held positions of responsibility. Perhaps this makes it all the harder to bear when PD robs them of their personal dignity and standing.

One other thing I would like to mention, even though I was given a bit of a brush off when I suggested it to the professionals. Near my home there are four houses in a road, two each side, almost opposite each other. Built, I think, before the war, in an unmade up road. In all four of them there are, or have been recently, people suffering from PD. This seems really too much of a coincidence. Four people living in such close proximity - what can they have in common? The only thing that I can think of is water pipes. If the pipes were made of - or fastened with - something that became toxic when water with all its present additives flowed through the pipes - could that have triggered off the PD?

I say triggered off, for I believe that in many people PD is latent, low-lying, until illness, trauma or some other stressful event allows it to develop at a much faster rate. Like a grenade waiting for the pin to be pulled out.

Recently I have been contacted by six sufferers or carers all living in three connected streets. Is this because:-

    (a)   They all have the same doctor and he or she has told them about us?
    (b)   There is something local causing people to get PD?
    (c)   They know each other and our name has been passed round as being helpful.

Are registers kept of how many PD sufferers there are in a practice? Do doctors have to notify anyone? If they did and it was given to some statisticians to work through, it might throw up some interesting information. It might also encourage the Health Councils to be more aware of the needs of sufferers and carers - their need of speech therapy, home care, etc.

It might even, wonder's breath indrawn, encourage them to set up some training of medical and professional staff in the vagaries and understanding of PD and the urgent need of help for the carers.

WHAT ABOUT A CURE?

At present there is sadly no cure. Those with a medical background (or who have learnt First Aid) will know that if brain cells die they cannot be replaced. So if the cells in the part of the brain that is affected by PD die, they are irreplaceable.

It is of very great importance to find out why these brain cells do start to die, and there are many research programmes going on.

If once a possible cure is found, or better still a way of identifying potential PD sufferers in advance, and so preventing the disease, there will still have to be many more years of research and testing to ensure that these new methods have no harmful side effects.

A cure, if found and carefully tested, could then be introduced. But will it ever be possible to replace dead brain cells? And of course prevention will only benefit the young unless, that is, it is found that our present belief that PD is present and active in the body for a long time before it becomes apparent, is found to be wrong.

At the time of writing researchers have just discovered that a certain drug used by HIV positive people is not the wonder drug they had thought it to be. Alas! There are many false dawns in research and great care has to be taken to test new drugs. Even then tragedies like the Thalidomide affair can happen. So it must be years yet before anything can be proved to be of use. We must look therefore to caring for and helping today's sufferers who are unlikely to benefit by any wonder drug.

HOW IS PD FIRST NOTICED

It is probably the sufferer who first actually mentions a problem. But it may be that other signs have been noticed and accepted as part of a person for years by the nearest and dearest, without realising that they are the early effects of PD. And it may be quite a long time after that before their doctor is involved.

A great friend of mine tells me that she had never seen her husband swing his arms when he was walking. She had just accepted this as part of him. His PD was not diagnosed until some five years after they were married.

PD may first appear as a slight dragging of one foot, or an inability to grip something properly; writing may get smaller, a face may lose its expression (or it may always have been a *poker face*), people may become easily tired, appear to be run down, or they move and respond more slowly. Sometimes a person may start to stoop, or their stoop may become more pronounced and will therefore be noticed ('hold your head up, you are really beginning to look old') and they may find it difficult to start or continue a movement or to get up out of a chair. Forgetfulness can be another sign; absent-mindedness or not quite with it. They may start to trip or fall (sometimes backwards).

But it is not a sudden obvious happening, it is not like someone coming out in a rash or having a broken leg. At first it may be a series of small inconveniences, occasional happenings. It may be put down to tiredness, to a rucked up carpet, to a 'bad day at the office'. No-one would say 'I have tripped over the carpet again, I must have Parkinson's'. Despite all our publicity efforts, people (and that includes many trained people I am sorry to say) may not know about or not understand PD. It is so varied, such a casual condition, only the person themselves would be able to clock up all the unusual things that have now started to happen to them and the very PD itself may inhibit such careful thought. Life today is too busy to think about oneself all the time. And anyhow, it might be caused by the uneven pavement or perhaps they are going a bit deaf? ('Yes, all right, next time I see the doctor I'll ask him').

So it may be for quite another reason that they see their doctor; a good family doctor who has known his patient for some time will pick up the signs of PD and may send him or her for further tests. His questions may cause the family to look back over the years and realise that things haven't been right for some time.

Of course there is the shake, with which people generally associate Parkinson's, but it is not necessarily present, it may be only internal. I have met several people who have had an internal tremor for some years, but have never thought of mentioning it to anyone.

The other day I looked at a Prayer Book given to me by my grandmother when I was seven, a very long time ago. I looked where she had written my name 'With love from her Grandmother'. Her handwriting just shouted 'Parkinson's' at me. Now she had died during the war, having become ill, and finished her life in a Nursing Home. I had never known what was wrong with her; I had just been told that she had drifted away from the world. But here was her crabbed handwriting, getting smaller and rising at the end of the line - a perfect example of a Parkinsonian's writing. There is no doubt in my mind now why she had 'drifted away'. But in those days I do not think people knew so much about PD, nor were there the drugs to help her.

There is one type of Parkinson's person to which there are many pointers. Whether they are like this because they have PD (even if it has not yet been diagnosed) or whether they are the sort of person that PD will attack I do not know. You may well know someone like this although no mention of PD has ever been mooted. Often their life has been saddened by a tragedy, they may have lost their loved partner or another member of the family and gradually they will have become lonely, shy, not wanting to go out much, and certainly not into crowded places. They will resist being organised, simply not co-operating. They may not like wide open spaces, or being shut in small rooms, or being driven at speed in a car. They may retreat into themselves when people speak too loudly to them. They may withdraw more into themselves as they get older.

You may see them shuffling quietly along the street, with their knees slightly bent, and their heads low. Although they may long for a bit of companionship, they want to be left alone to carry on their restricted lives. They really are not Day Centre fodder. They may be classified by busy people as 'not a good mixer'. In fact they may just want to be left alone; they are sensitive to noise and bustle and, as their (undiagnosed?) PD develops and things become more difficult, their personal hygiene may get out of control (the bodily functions can change quite a bit). Most cruel and damning of all, neighbours and friends may say they are 'not a bit like the rest of the family'.

Because there is no one sign always present which 'outsiders' can recognise, there can be a lot of misunderstanding, criticism or even bullying. And if people do not realise that something is wrong they can make very hurtful remarks, which can make a sufferer's life even worse, and that of the carer. The family of someone who has been in a car crash will get lots of sympathetic help. A deaf or a blind person can also be recognised (if only by their delightful Guide Dog or their earpiece). Deafness and blindness is understood, quite naturally spoken of and accepted by friends and neighbours. Their faces are expressive and their body movement normal and under control. There is no embarrassment in being with a blind or deaf person but if the person's body movements are bizarre and unnatural things can be very different.

On the other hand many PD people, when they are seen outside their homes on a good day, do not appear to have anything wrong with them at all, and the friends and neighbours may wonder what all the fuss is about. But on a bad day, when the body is out of control, then things can go very wrong. I must admit that if I saw a man or woman weaving up the street I might think 'drink' rather than 'PD' - that is to say I would have before I knew about PD.

The family may know little about PD before it is diagnosed, and they, too, may feel it is rather weird and may even try to hide it from their neighbours and friends. A shaking hand will be thrust into a pocket or a shopping trolley will be used to steady the walk. The partner will work hard to keep up a front, even after diagnosis. But friendships may wither and die. Food often gets spilt, and then they are thought to be keeping themselves to themselves because now that the hand has become shaky and clothes stained they do not wish to go out to meals.

There are many such sad cases of misunderstanding. A friend of mine confessed to me that her neighbours had told their children not to go into her house any more 'in case it was catching', and another told me that she was told by some new arrivals in their road that her husband 'ought to be put away' because it was not nice to have him where their children could see him 'and bad for the neighbourhood'.

Those close to an early Parkinsonian may not notice any changes, because PD usually develops slowly and if a person is elderly the changes may well be put down to their age. But friends and relations coming to visit after a period of six months or longer, may be very shocked. Children may be devastated by the sight of a stooped and shaking father or mother, and may blame the partner for not telling them or for not going to the doctor. Distress is eased if someone can be blamed.

WHAT BRINGS PD OUT INTO THE OPEN?

Any extra stress is liable to weaken resistance to the progress of PD and the condition will then become more noticeable and distressing. I would say that PD may become worse, more tiresome and more obvious after any of the following emotional shocks or body problems:-

A moment of deep emotion, sadness, fear, distress, the death of someone they love;

A moment of personal embarrassment or social stress. (Some time ago I saw a man threatened on TV. A fist was thrust in his face and he was shouted at in front of other people. His face remained expressionless, his body did not flinch and his voice remained quiet and colourless. There was just no response. Did he have PD?);

An accident, a serious injury, a moment of great danger or stress. ('He was allowed home, but he was never quite the same person');

An operation, a period away from home in strange surroundings and without the family around; this might have frightened the sufferer, distressed or embarrassed. Does the emotional stress of going into hospital cause PD to develop or is it the medication, the operation or the anaesthetic? Several times I have been told that X went into hospital for a minor operation but 'caught his Parkinson's when he was in'.

If we are right that people have PD for a long time before it shows outwardly, e.g. they may already be <u>affected</u> by it, but not in any physically recognisable way, then when they suffer some severe shock or trauma the PD may come out into the open, taking a greater hold of the sufferer's body and becoming much more disabling and distressing. This may well make the family think that it was 'caught' in hospital.

Of course ageing also allows PD to get a stronger grip, but I would say that stress plays the largest part in the development of PD.

SOME OUTWARD SIGNS OF PD?

There are many signs of PD that will be picked up by those experienced in the condition. Sometimes one can recognise PD in someone on the TV or in the way they speak on the radio, or pictured in a newspaper, and of course one often sees a probable Parkinsonian in the street.

Never, ever, should one think of PD as a condition where the problems are always the same, either in two sufferers or in one sufferer on <u>two consecutive days</u>. And never, ever, compare one PD sufferer's behaviour against that of another's. 'Oh I don't think Mr L really has Parkinson's; we used to have a Mr K here and he had Parkinson's and he never did that'.

We should take an individual interest in an individual's particular needs and problems. I have heard someone say 'It would be nice for Mr P to come here on Tuesdays and Thursdays. They are the days Mr Q comes and he has Parkinson's and they could sit together'. Lucky they did not arrange for all the one-legged men to come on the same day and sit together!

A neighbour of ours had a hand tremor (both visible and something you could feel inside of her hand if she held yours). This was never mentioned, just accepted as part of her, although I know that I, for one, did not like it. I think we just thought of her, on the strength of the tremor, as highly strung and excitable. But when she was over eighty she was diagnosed as having Parkinson's. Perhaps it is of interest to mention that she was very ill while she was a nurse just behind the French Front Line during the First World War. She was unwell for a long time and eventually was told that there was one doctor who knew the cure for her trouble. But he was German, feeling still ran very high and she could not bring herself to go to him.

A few years later she had a 'nervous breakdown' after she had locked herself into an attic by mistake when she was alone in a house in London. She was there for nearly a day before being rescued. If she had latent PD then nothing could have been worse for her. She never did really recover her strength or health and this experience brought on a form of claustrophobia as well. But she was one of the most active and outgoing people I know so maybe the PD was still under control. It was not until she was eighty in about 1977 when she was too infirm to live on her own that she was diagnosed as having PD by the Rest Home doctor.

See next page for some of the outward signs of PD:-

- Tremor of hands, head, arms, legs (and it may be the thighs, not the lower legs);

- Sudden inability to continue a movement already started, such as walking; or someone may only be able to walk backwards, not forwards, or be able to climb stairs but not walk forward;

- Slowness with any ordinary movement, drinking, swallowing, turning the body, getting out of a chair, moving the eyes, starting to speak (after that the speed of speech will probably increase greatly and become a sort of rapid mumble or fluttery waffle);

- Great tiredness (not sleepiness), lassitude or a 'wet rag' feeling so that it becomes more and more difficult to initiate anything;

- No arm swing, and pain in shoulders and arms, often described as rheumatism or arthritis;

- Weakness of the back with an increasing stoop, and loss of upright position. I know of a Day Centre where they say all their PD people sleep a lot in their nice warm, airless sitting room after lunch. But if you go up and look at them you may well see that they are wide awake but their backs have given out and so their bodies have slouched down onto the tables in front of them. Because their speech is poor and slow and quiet, and their thought process may be slow also, they do not manage to draw someone's attention to ask for a pull up again. But it would be better if they could, for then they could see what was going on and join in some of the activities;

- Dragging one leg;

- Walking as though they were slightly sitting down. Their knees are a little bent and seem to be ahead of the rest of their body, and their hands are often forward too, a little like a dog begging;

- Alternatively, they shuffle along with their body bent as though their head was being pulled down and the rest of the body following in a gentle curve. This may well get progressively worse;

- Loss of smile and face expression;

- Feet 'glued to the floor' or juddering on the spot. I think that this is the result of trying to get going but that the signal coming through from the brain is too weak to do more than lift the feet up and down on the spot - no forward movement. My car sometimes loses power in this sort of way;

- You will be thinking that I have forgotten the obvious contortions of the body and distortions of the face (they are *not* facial expressions). I have not forgotten - who could? - but I think everyone knows about them. What perhaps they have not thought about is that these dreadful endless contortions are extremely tiring and distressing and have to be lived with every day. Unless sufferers tell us, how can we know what they feel about all this?

And that bring me to the next section.

BODY LANGUAGE

I am glad that you have read so far, as we now come to something of paramount importance - and which often leads to great misunderstanding - in the care of people with PD.

There are two sorts of Body Language to consider in relation to PD. The normal, natural, understandable body language and the other sort: PD Body Language.

<u>Understandable Body Language</u>

It must be very difficult for a blind person to gauge someone's reactions. For half our communication comes from the expressions on our faces. Smiles, frowns, opening our eyes wide. Someone who is blind must have to listen very carefully to the tone of voice to know how a person is responding to their conversation.

Just try saying 'Look out, the house is on fire' and you will realise how much of what you are saying is enhanced and developed by the movements of your face and body. The first time a baby smiles is a moment of tremendous joy to its parents. It <u>responded</u> to them and it is therefore mentally active and in communication. And children and adults use their faces all the time to express their feelings. We smile, wink, screw up our eyes, raise our eyebrows (a good way, I was told, to express fatigue on the stage). Children stand in front of the mirror and get the giggles making up odd faces. Face expression is 60 or 70 per cent of communication. (Think of the person in the telephone box ahead of you; you can almost tell what they are saying and their relationship to the person they are speaking to, even though you can hear nothing).

Your face also sends out messages that you do not know about. 'Don't frown' someone will say. A child will know you are cross and at the end of your tether when he sees your lips tighten up. Just watch people waiting at the exit from the customs shed when a plane has been delayed. As their traveller comes through the door the whole of their body as well as their faces sends out a message of relief and happiness.

And think how heartrending it is to see an adult breaking down in tears.

Your body sends out other messages also. Fingers drumming, feet tapping, holding out your arms to a child, waving someone goodbye, covering your face with your hands in sorrow or distress, a child jigging up and down with excitement. These are all silent messages which will be noticed, read <u>and responded to</u> by any other person present. And often if you see an adult in tears it will be very difficult not to respond by crying yourself.

<u>PD Body Language</u>

There is only one message sent out in PD Body Language. This message is *'I am a sufferer of PD. I am not always able to control my face or body movements. Please ignore anything bizarre or unnatural, and please do not be distressed or offended by anything the PD makes my body do or prevents it doing'*.

There are four sections to this that you will need to be aware of:-

1   The No-Body-Language

Some types of PD cause the sufferer to lose almost all ability to communicate with the body for part or all of the day. A smile is seldom seen, the body does not respond to any emotion. When you put your arm round them - and I hope you will go on giving your sufferer lots of love - you will get little or no response, although the emotion may increase PD effects. You will not be able to read his or her thoughts by the expression on their face or the movement of the body. A rider to this is that if a visitor calls the visit could stimulate the sufferer into greater ability for a short time, which can be hard on the carer who has had no response all day and then sees a partner responding to a stranger.

There is another twist to the No-Body-Language: if the sufferer has no body language people will not recognise any change in the mental or bodily condition. They will not know if the sufferer is amused by a joke, animated by any news or tired. If someone is tired it normally shows by a strained look on the face or by the body movements, but not so with the PD sufferer. 'Dad always shakes, sometimes more than others' so Dad may not get the extra consideration and support that a fit person would get if _they_ looked tired or unhappy.

2   The Bizarre Body Language

Everybody knows about this, but I wonder whether many people realise how tiring as well as embarrassing and inhibiting it must be for the sufferer. And remember he cannot hide himself away during his writhing attacks nor can his face show his embarrassment. In public, among friends, he will see that they are, perhaps, more embarrassed for themselves than they are for him.

And at home what do the children think? And what does the sufferer feel about the children being present while his PD is forcing him to writhe and make odd faces? What, he may wonder, will the children's friends think - and will the children still want to bring their friends home?

How true it is that PD affects the life and social standing of the whole family.

Incidentally, did you know that people can also suffer from an internal tremor? It is seldom mentioned by sufferers because they do not realise you do not know about it (an open secret?) and as it is only inside them they do not have to explain anything to their friends; but if you should casually mention that some people suffer in this way you will often get an immediate response. 'Oh, I have that. It is very distressing, you don't know. It never stops'.

I once mentioned this to someone, who I thought knew all about PD. Her reaction greatly shocked me. She said 'Oh, I don't suppose she really does shake internally. She probably just said that to get your sympathy'. What an attitude from a nurse.

Her remark was one of the reasons why I am writing this booklet.

3   USBL (Unsocial Body Language)

Sorry to mention this. Dribbling, food-stained clothes (so often on the most fastidious people), unattractive scalp and face blemishes, sometimes flaking off onto clothes, even poor hygiene may all be due to the PD and not to 'letting themselves go'. They must hate all this as much as it disgusts others. I am very ashamed to think that I sometimes find it difficult to give my PD friends a big hug because of their USBL.

Baths must be something PD sufferers miss out on due to the difficulty of getting in and out. Good Nursing Homes and Respite Care and Residential Homes do invest in the wonder baths that enable a disabled person once more to enjoy a proper bath. I believe that if someone invested in a few of these special baths for the disabled and called themselves a Bathette (like a Laundrette) many people would rise up and called them blessed. Maybe there could even be a travelling Bathette that would go to people's homes or maybe the Hospital Trusts could consider installing a number of such baths which could be used through the day and evening. I would like to think that members of the St John Ambulance and Red Cross could be used in this connection. I do know of one Day Centre where such a system is run by the Centre with the help of volunteers. It must come, surely. Perhaps we had better work on it ourselves. How about a legacy from someone? Or what about the special bath manufacturers wading in?

Hair washing, too, is very important. This is because some of the PD medication causes excessive sweating and the sweat may remain on the scalp and hair and make a person unattractive to be near.

I was surprised to hear from a nursing friend that one of her PD patients was scrupulously particular about his hygiene, insisting on daily baths and hair washing. I used to take him out in the evenings sometimes and I found his body odour, and the odour from his scalp, very trying. Although he has now moved away I am glad to be able to remember him with more respect.

Washing can often be helped by the wonderful helpers who will come in to help get a person up in the morning. But they are overworked and I know of one husband who has had to dispense with their services because their timing was so varied that he found it difficult to plan his wife's medication, so that she was 'unlocked' at the time when they came. Medication takes about half an hour to work through on PD people, so if the helper was late or early she would find the person was not in a state that she could be helped. This, of course, was a particularly bad case.

But how awful it must be for husband and wife who have always had a good standing in their neighbourhood and workplace to <u>know</u> that one of them is now bodily unattractive and that people find it difficult to visit them. And perhaps I might add in this connection that dedicated carers do not always realise how 'stuffy' a room or house will become if their sufferer is always in one room and kept warm by a gas or electric fire with little or no ventilation. As they are in it all the time they will not notice the unpleasant atmosphere, but oh my goodness! some houses require a real effort to go into.

A sideline to USBL is that it may prevent a problem being properly attended to. A friend of mine who lives in a caring establishment was told he could no longer eat with the other residents because 'his manners were so poor and his eating habits unattractive'. In future he must take his meals in his own room. And so he was wheeled back to his bedroom and his meal set down beside him. The manager then told me that this poor chap had lost his temper and thrown his food about his room! What a shattering example of misunderstanding in a person running a caring establishment. I think the Manager really should have known that the sufferer had not the strength in his limbs, nor the control, to do such a thing. Nor, he should have known, was he the sort of person who would want to do so.

What had actually happened was that without the inspiration of being with other people (which often improves a person's PD for a short time), and shattered by his fellow residents' rejection of him, this poor man had tried in vain to feed himself. But his inability to grasp his knife and fork and guide them to his mouth had become even worse under the stress of the degradation which he had suffered, and his <u>tremor</u> became a <u>flap</u>. When I called he was still struggling to get a mouthful into his mouth and to make it worse 'the kitchen' came in and said they must take his tray now, as they went off at two. He was <u>not</u> angry; he was sad, distressed, shamed and very hungry. How could people be so callous to a fellow human being afflicted with PD?

Of course feeding and pleasant behaviour is a must in such an establishment; I am only saying that the matter should have been managed in a much more tactful manner. And when anyone can take hold of your wheelchair and wheel you away just as if you were a baby ... awful.

4. <u>The OK Body Language</u>

A happier subject to end this section on. But still there is a misunderstood message. Carers, caring partners, will always try to turn their partner out as best they may, especially when they have an appointment to see a doctor or go to a clinic or Day Centre. They may even adjust their medication for the day so that the sufferer is at their best and most mobile during the period away from home. <u>But this can backfire</u>. For people will see the sufferer coping comparatively well, and make remarks such as 'she makes too much fuss of him', 'he is quite all right when he is with me, she does too much for him' and even the one about making a cane for their own back. We <u>are</u> inclined to make light of our problems when we see the doctor or dentist, in the hope that they will agree with us that there is not much wrong, and the doctor himself may not realise the extent of the problem if he only sees a sufferer when they are well enough to come to the surgery, or have had their medication adjusted by their carer so that they are physically easier to manage while out of the house.

It is only too easy, when one has a busy programme, to accept the appearance and condition of the sufferer as he or she appears at that moment. PD sufferers are the sort of people it is very easy to - I was going to say bully, but it is not that. It is more that one can override their complaints. I am so often told that a carer has been told 'Well I can get you an appointment to see X or Y, but I don't honestly think there is anything more that can be done. I've done all that is possible'. But PD is a deep and devious condition with many, many different facets and forms, and the condition can vary from minute to minute. Stress, as you know, often makes a person worse but conversely someone can be hyped up by seeing someone different or when in an unusual (but friendly) situation. They often suffer for it later, though.

Another problem with OK Body Language is that when the sufferer is seen again by their doctor or consultant a few months later and is obviously worse there may be a suggestion that 'this is just a bad day; he should not have deteriorated so much in such a short time'. In other words, he will be judged against his 'good' day last time, as not too badly afflicted, just bad luck he is having a bad day today, and the correct message, that he is deteriorating and it was just good luck he was seen on a good day, will not be received. And the carer will not be given the extra help that he or she now needs so badly.

This can also be the case if he was 'ON' last time and this time, when the appointment is, say, in the afternoon and not the morning, he is having an 'OFF'. (You will read more about 'OFF' and 'ON' later).

And yet another problem. Nurses and doctors are <u>trained</u>, they may feel they know it all. They may even criticise the carer and bully her into believing she is over anxious, over caring, over working for the sufferer. I believe the professionals need to take great care to approach all families with PD in a very humble way, learning from them rather than judging them. The carer, <u>on their own very often</u>, has kept the sufferer going till now, at home with only spasmodic help. It is seldom, I believe, that a nurse or doctor or consultant are alone in a clinic, there must always be helpers around, so how can they judge what it is like to cope with a heavy person with little movement <u>on their own</u>, and throughout the day and night? To have their daily grind underestimated, even criticised, is not going to help anyone and may even cause the carer (and sufferer) to lose faith in the professionals. I do not believe that sort of attitude, nor the 'Oh well, you aren't too bad really, are you?' approach to be good 'caring'. Medication is only a part of caring for PD - the real caring is at home, the often single-handed caring by an elderly partner, day and night.

TO SUM UP

Let me ask you a question. If you were ill, do you think your character would change, would you become more difficult to care for, vindictive, spiteful, slothful, make things harder for those who help you? Would you be able to keep up such a nasty character so foreign to your nature? Would you dribble, spill your food, stare with expressionless face, be too late at the loo, just to add to the difficulties that your partner was coping with? Would you decide to do all this just to annoy?

What a really stupid question. Of course you wouldn't - if for no other reason than that you depend on them too much. Why, then, do people so often blame the sufferer for what PD causes his body to do?

Could it be because they have not had the time to think it through? Have they been taught badly, perhaps, or absorbed the attitudes of old-fashioned nurses? Been 'warned' about PD sufferers and told not to let them get away with it?

Or could it be that it is so strange, so unaccountable, so changeable in different sufferers, so bizarre, and without any body language, that it is easier to criticise the carer - or even the sufferer - than try to understand and cope with this insidious and horrid condition of Parkinson's Disease?

ON/OFF AND ITS PROBLEMS

This effect of PD must have a section all to itself; it is very important indeed and needs careful consideration. It is so important that I always write it in capital letters. ON/OFF.

ON/OFF is seen mostly, I am told, in people who have been on medication for a long time and it follows that people who are well served by their medication will need to keep scrupulously to the proper timing or, as the effects wear off, they may go OFF and become poorly. It is therefore important that PD sufferers always carry a signed card from their doctor authorising the somewhat unusual timing of their medication, and that carers are very careful that the sufferers take enough medication with them when they go out and that someone is warned of the time medication is due. And that like diabetics, sufferers may use up their medication more quickly on occasion and may not realise this or be able to ask for help.

ON/OFF has social as well as medical implications. If someone you know quite well suddenly ignores you, does not respond to your greeting at all, you are liable to feel snubbed, even to take offence, especially if this happens in front of others. If the behaviour is different from the way you were treated last week you may think the sufferer is being awkward, surly or putting it on, even being downright rude.

But this can easily happen; and it can be sudden and unexpected. At a meeting with sufferers from PD I once saw a man sitting with a number of doctors on a platform quite suddenly go OFF. The doctors did not notice; it was a lay person who saw what had happened and hastened to give him his medication. But why had they missed it?

Whatever their medication, sufferers are differently affected at different times of the day. A man I greatly admire and whose wife has dedicated her life to caring for him, can make miniatures and tiny trains for a model railway, join thin wires together, screw tiny screws, in the morning, but is helpless, stiff and demanding in the afternoon. His brain is very active, which possibly increases his problems as he is unable to 'let go' during his bad times. He appears to worry a great deal about his breathing during the OFF period, which after all is an instinctive fear in all of us. (Put your head under the blankets for a minute or two. See how quickly you bring your head out when you have used up all the oxygen! Remember what it was like being winded when playing games at school and how you fought for breath).

Unfortunately, because of the wide variance in his behaviour - the nurses call it 'his moods' which of course it isn't - he is labelled selfish, naughty, tiresome, difficult, rude, time wasting, everything under the sun that blames <u>him</u> for his behaviour and not his PD. If only we could get this home to people, if <u>only</u> they could see that it is the PD taking over and not him I think his life would be happier.

We do not blame a man who has had a stroke if he cannot write his name clearly, nor do we blame a deaf man if he cannot hear what we say, or a blind man if he cannot see where he is going. Why then, oh why do we blame PD sufferers for the way their PD causes them to behave? Is it lack of training? Or is it lack of sympathy? Or is it because PD people cannot speak for themselves and may not even realise what is happening to them? Is it because there is often no obvious, recognisable sign or symptom, the person appearing complete but slow? Is it, oh dear, because they are vulnerable and weak and they may take a moment or two to answer, and then in a low voice, or may not respond to requests or orders and so they get bullied?

I have heard people say '<u>We</u> don't let them sleep when they are here; we keep them awake and give them lots of stimulating things to do'. Fine - but what do you think the poor sufferer is like by the time he or she gets home, if the normal routine has been upset (which will cause stress - more about that later)? Please remember the reason you have a PD sufferer in a Day Centre or Hospital is <u>to reduce the pressure at home</u>. Therefore it is the condition of the person when they arrive home that matters above everything else.

We cannot tell what a sufferer thinks about all this for he or she may no longer be well enough to be asked or to reply to such disturbing questions. However we should try to remember that PD families are not in a position to make new friends and may come to rely very heavily on old ones. Please do not withdraw your friendship when PD strikes a family you know. They will need you more and more.

Things taught or achieved do not last long with a bad case of PD; the thing to aim at when caring for someone with PD is lack of stress, worry, fear, so that the condition does not get worse. Keep the person ticking over in the comfortable, easy, usual way that they can rely on. That way you will earn their - and even more, their carer's - affection, gratitude and <u>trust</u>.

Phrases to avoid when caring for a Parkinsonian:-

She can't expect...

We have other people to look after, you know...

When Mr X was here he was able to...

He must fit into OUR routine...

I have only one pair of legs, you know (but at least they can be used, someone with PD may not be able to move at all)...

It doesn't really matter about the time of his medicine - let him have his when the others have theirs...

SOME PD PROBLEMS

1. <u>Depression</u>

This is an *in* word among people working with Parkinson's sufferers and their families. I have given a great deal of thought to this word 'depression', and I still believe it is over-used or even possibly wrongly used.

If someone with full control over speech and body language said they were depressed, and looked it, I would agree that they were depressed. They were able to tell us that that was what they were feeling. But I think we can misread the feelings of a PD sufferer and take the <u>No-Body-Language</u> as actually being <u>Body Language</u>. I do not see how you can say someone is depressed just because you are getting no messages from him. If someone does not smile we should not say that he is intentionally <u>not</u> smiling, i.e. is depressed. He may think he is smiling, he may be sending out the right message from his brain, but it is not getting through. But because his face can no longer give the message of cheerfulness we should not say he is depressed. Because he cannot react to OUR body language, our smiles and cheerful chat, we should not say that he is rejecting them. We should realise that it is his <u>PARKINSON'S</u>, not he, that is blocking his natural reaction, or distorting the message he wants to send. His body can no longer speak for him.

It is interesting that after a person has had a stroke he is said to 'express emotion easily', that is to say, his eyes may fill with tears which run down his cheeks. This is, in fact, the person being deprived by his stroke of his normal 'stiff upper lip' control. It is embarrassing; we do not like to see a grown man cry. But once more we should realise that it is not he, so much, as the breakdown in the normal functional control of his body.

In PD this is reversed; we say someone is looking depressed because his body and speech <u>are not displaying any emotion whatever</u>. His body is no longer able to display what he is feeling or to be used to enhance conversation. Indeed it may be almost impossible for him to speak, and very often if he does speak it is garbled, or too quick, unclear or very, very soft. But none of that inability is positively saying 'I am depressed'. The message, if there is one, is surely 'At present I cannot communicate'. Many PD sufferers 'just sit there, staring in front of them making no effort to talk or smile'. How do we know they are making no effort? How dare we accuse them of making no effort. How do we know that they are depressed? You might as well say that a person standing in the dark is depressed because you cannot see him smiling! And, Heaven help us, this poor sufferer may think he <u>is</u> smiling and is wondering why no-one is smiling back. Why, he may be thinking, are they all looking so depressed <u>when I am smiling at them</u>?

So go on, whether you get a smile back or not, whether he speaks or not, whether his body is stiff or moving disjointedly or shaking, keep cheerful, keep caring, keep including him in the conversation, keep giving all Parkinsonians the respect, the friendship and the cheerfulness they so badly need. Members of St John Ambulance speak of those who need their help as 'Our Masters the Sick'. We should think of Parkinsonians, and their carers, in this way.

2. Hallucinations

Some sufferers who have been on their medication a long time suffer from hallucinations. They see rabbits, Indian girls, firemen or snakes; but whatever it is, it is far more of a nuisance, I think, for the carer than it is for the sufferer. How would you cope if your partner started to swear there was a snake under the bed or if they started having conversations with a little Indian girl? Or what if they saw a camel plodding along the garden path - how would you cope? Would you go along with his hallucination and 'see' them too? Or would you say 'You're hallucinating, don't do it?' I do not myself know what the right approach is. But whatever you did you would be upset, distressed and even worrying about your partner's sanity.

It is up to the outside carer to find out from the partner early on whether the sufferer has periods of hallucinating and how they wish you to respond to them. They may themselves need counselling about this. It is difficult to act a lie and this can lead to friction and more problems. But it is equally difficult to say to a person of strong character that they are hallucinating. Please be on the lookout for this problem and take advice from the carer and others, but chiefly from the carer, because your actions may affect both partners, and if unsatisfactory may lead to the cancellation of further visits.

And be very careful not to spread any rumours about little Indian girls, firemen or snakes ... it is all too easy for something like that to become misreported and cause still further distress to the carer.

Whatever you think or believe, please be guided by the carer in your reaction and behaviour. They will have to go on dealing with the situation long after you have gone home, and over the months they have decided how they wish to deal with it to help their partner and themselves.

PS: The other day I visited a sufferer and his family; he did not know that hallucination could be part of the PD pattern; the relief on his face when I mentioned it was worth everything. 'I had not dared to speak about it to anyone, not even my wife or doctor' he said. 'I truly thought I might be going mad and would have to go into a home'. Another reason/justification for writing this booklet.

3. Swallowing

Loss of full control over the tongue will cause several problems; slurred speech and slowness in eating and swallowing among them. And of course the latter will probably lead to loss of weight. In fact I usually know when these problems start because there is quite suddenly the beginning of a bowed and cadaverous appearance. The face becomes bony and clothes begin to hang on the body. The carer, not understanding, may complain that the sufferer is 'picking at his food', 'won't eat and won't take his medicine', or even 'just holds his pills in his mouth and won't swallow them' without understanding the true cause.

Of course hearing these sorts of comments will again increase the stress and therefore make things more difficult. But let us take this a bit further and think of the actual mechanics of eating, something we haven't had to <u>think</u> about since the days of childhood when we were learning to control spoons and forks. For if the Parkinsonian is going downhill he will have to think about, and try to initiate a number of activities with different parts of his body before the food is safely in his stomach. You may get a little bit of the feel of his difficulties by trying to eat your meal with your knife or spoon in your left hand and a very big fork in your right.

To eat a meal you have to get to the table and be sitting the right way round at the right height. Food which you may or may not like will be set down in front of you, to eat, whether you are hungry or not, whether your mouth is dry or full of saliva, whether your medication makes you feel nauseous or not. You must then grip a spoon or knife and fork and, controlling your shake and trying to guide your wayward hand towards your plate, you must take the food onto the fork or spoon and then turn the implement round and, without dropping any of it and without your arm suddenly jerking out away from your body, you must guide the food into your mouth, which must have been opened at just the right time and be where you thought it was. At this moment you will find out whether the food is too hot or too dry or too salty to enjoy. The spoon or fork must then be withdrawn from your closed mouth and your hand and arm guided back towards the plate.

You may be able to stop for a minute then, or you may be encouraged to start collecting up the next mouthful although your concentration is fully occupied in chewing what is in your mouth. But now comes the most difficult moment of all, for Parkinsonians lose much of their power over their tongues, and tongues are necessary to push the chewed food back towards the throat so that it may start its journey to the stomach. Often and often the food just cannot be got to the back of the mouth and a sufferer will sit with it in his mouth, unable to move it one way or the other. And while he is working hard at this final movement (and with a full mouth he cannot explain what is happening) he is hurried and hurried by people telling him to hurry up, and the rest of the food is slowing congealing on his plate.

And that is only the first mouthful.

The business of drinking is equally, or even more, fraught, for liquid can travel a long way if your hand shakes at the wrong time, and again it is very difficult to drink out of a shaking cup or suck up liquid through a straw. Many people lose the strength of suck needed when using a straw, although there is less danger of spills. I wonder if we cannot invent a gravity feeder, such as one uses in pets' cages, where the liquid seeps slowly down by gravity. This would at least mean that the sufferer did not have to suck <u>up</u> from a cup on a table some twelve inches below his face.

Try swallowing without using your tongue or with it clapped firm to the roof of your mouth. Try, in fact, what it is like to suffer some of the effects of Parkinson's.

NB: There is a glimmer of light here; very often if you can encourage a sufferer to take a drink of very cold water before a meal it will stimulate the swallow. Perhaps, also, a small cold compress placed on the cheek or below the jaw might have the same effect, but I have not tried that yet.

4. <u>Speech and Speech Therapy</u>

A friend of mine was told by the Speech Therapist in her area that sufferers from PD could not be helped to regain their speech, or to retain it, if they had 'allowed it to deteriorate too much'. They should, she was told, 'self refer' early on. This is an important point. You do not need a doctor's letter to ask for a speech assessment.

But it is also an interesting point. Early 'self referral' presumes that people know that something is beginning to go wrong and that there is a way of curing or lessening that wrong. But how many people, especially the elderly ones, know about speech therapy? And how many people with PD would realise that it is their speech that is failing and not that their partner is beginning to go deaf? As far as I know neither my husband nor I have Parkinson's. But _he_ complains that my speech is not so clear while _I_ am sure that it is his hearing that is less acute. We agree that there is something not so good with the other one, but never in a thousand years would it have occurred to either of us that I needed speech therapy (nor would we have known that I could 'self refer') which frankly - as there is nothing wrong with my speech - would I have thought of investigating it. I think I would regard it as a waste of NHS money, especially as it is not me but my husband who needs help. In fact I would have been trying to get him to go to a hard of hearing clinic. In a few years, if, in fact I have got PD but do not know it and my speech gets worse, it will be too late.

But once being seen by a Speech Therapist there are many other difficulties that such a therapist can help with; breathing, dribbling, etc. I have often thought that sufferers should be made much more conscious of the need to breathe deeply (and thus keep a good breathing ability) and that their rooms should be well ventilated with plenty of good fresh, oxygenated air.

So many homes I have visited have been 'nice and warm' (and really rather smelly) because the carer wants to keep the sufferer warm. I believe PD brains, even more than ordinary brains, need plenty of oxygen to keep them alert. A nice warm room often has poor ventilation so as not to 'waste the electricity'. But the result may be that the sufferer gets more and more comatose and the carer resents the way he sleeps so much. They should be warned about this.

Incidentally that goes for schools and offices too. None of the schools I pass, or visit, ever seems to have any windows open - nor do the offices. What they must smell like at the end of a working day I dread to think. If only people learnt of the importance of OXYGEN and of how it is used up with every breath anyone takes. People often seem to be kept warm yet starved of life-essential oxygen in Residential Care Homes and Nursing Homes. Architects do not seem to understand the importance of providing warmth _and_ ventilation.

There are homes I love to visit, not only for the welcome and friendliness, but also for the freshness and fragrance (and these are often the homes with doubly incontinent residents). But others - oh how I dread my visits. _I_ only have to be there for an hour or so; what must it be like to live there?

SUPPORTING SERVICES

It is sad that the different problems of PD have generally to be referred to different clinics or specialties and that there is no special clinic (other than the Romford Project) where all problems can be considered together. Constipation or swallowing, speech loss or low abdominal pain, rigidity or arthritic pain, tremor or 'depression', it would be good if a PD clinic could consider <u>all</u> the effects together and possibly give some information and practical advice to sufferers and carers as well.

The treatment prescribed for one effect of PD may sometimes be difficult to follow or even be inadvisable when other symptoms in the same patient are taken into account. For instance a person with a poor swallow may find it difficult to follow the suggested treatment for constipation.

Perhaps also Health Visitors could be offered an in-depth course on PD and its numerous and varied effects. So often PD sufferers are almost housebound. This may well mean that the carer is also, and therefore <u>they</u> need as much support as the sufferer. The strain of caring day and night with no break does not seem to be taken much into account by those who could most easily arrange for the burden to be eased.

But in this context I would like to make one point, about which I feel deeply. Sending a sufferer away for 'respite care' is not always the answer. Separation from their partner and home will often cause a great deal of stress, which can cause acceleration of the PD condition. It may also give the carer a feeling of guilt at sending their partner away. There is the further worry as to whether the partner's speech will be understood and the rigid programme of medication adhered to. Often the result is that the partner spends most of their time with their sufferer - causing some fairly sharp comments from those who do not understand. The best sort of 'respite care' for both is to send them off somewhere <u>together</u>; to somewhere where the burden of living and caring is taken off the carer, but they are still together so that there is no stress.

There is a holiday flat attached to a geriatric hospital in Cambridge where a couple can spend a fortnight or so with every sort of help in nursing etc, put in by the excellent Hospital, but quite separate from it. Really good catering is provided also by the Hospital, and there are also cooking facilities in the flat. The arrangements for this flat are made by a really kind and sympathetic person, who has become a friend of all those who have stayed there. Speech therapy, night nursing and turning etc, can all be arranged. Almost all the people who have stayed there have come back for another break. To me <u>this</u> is the way to give respite care without causing the stress and difficulties so often experienced (but seldom reported) when sufferers go away on their own where strangers may not understand or keep to the familiar routine.

As always with any illness or distressing condition we must think what would be the most helpful and valuable respite for the carer, and try to provide <u>that</u>, instead of presuming to 'know what is good for them' and taking the initiative away from those we think we are helping. Any unfavourable remarks made by the carer afterwards should be carefully considered and not dismissed as ungrateful or grumbling. The carer can tell us so much if we will only listen.

It has been suggested that trained helpers could stay in a sufferer's own home, taking the work off the shoulders of the carer who would still be there to ensure that the sufferer is properly cared for and understood. But that needs a lot of careful experiment before it can be offered to those who need it most. So much depends on personalities.

The final judgment on all respite care must surely be '<u>Are the sufferer and carer going to be better and derive long term benefit from the break, or has it created more problems?</u>' We, the outsiders, can never know best. We <u>must</u> listen and be prepared to learn and adjust our ideas to the needs that are expressed by those we want to help. Never must we allow ourselves to say, as I heard someone say once, 'Well, what did she expect? A free holiday? She asked for a break and that is exactly what she got. She can't expect everything'. Someone who is caring for a partner twenty-four hours a day, seven days a week, fifty-two weeks in the year, watching the decline of the partner they love <u>does</u> deserve everything, and it should be our pride and pleasure to try to provide what <u>they</u> want. We should not dictate, we should listen, learn and strive to provide.

TREATMENT OF SUFFERERS FROM PARKINSON'S DISEASE

There are many ways in which PD can be 'held', or rather the effects of PD can be held if a careful routine of medication is worked out and strictly followed.

Carers become very expert at his; they recognise the various ways in which PD affects their sufferer and they learn to give the right medication at exactly the right time. They are the ones who really KNOW. And it is they, of course who would normally have problems if this regime was not adhered to. It is hard for 'outsiders' to understand the importance of sticking rigidly to the timing and dosage or to realise what will happen if this plan is upset. Even doctors looking after people in respite care homes will sometimes 'up' the dosage without proper consideration of the effects. This may cause carers to say they will 'never let X go <u>there</u> again'.

As with diabetics, a Parkinsonian suffers greatly from stress if he is not confident that he will receive his medication at the right time, and the effects of his medication can cease as unexpectedly as a diabetic's can. Most hospitals and nursing homes are very careful with diabetics, for the result of wrongly timed medication can be dramatic and damaging. Not so many professional people realise how finely balanced is the timing of the medication of a Parkinsonian. And if the medication is not strictly adhered to the PD may become so much worse that he is unable to tell the nurses what is wrong; and then they, seeing that he is in a bad way think that he is not to be trusted to control his own medication and the situation whirls into a downward spiral of distress and suffering. Until a diabetic goes hypo he is vocal and reasonable, and there will be physical signs that something is wrong, but it may not be thus with a Parkinsonian whose body may become more and more silent and rigid if the drug regime is upset.

A carer made an interesting point to me the other day. I do not know if others have found the same thing. PD medication sometimes makes a person <u>worse</u> for the first half hour. It is therefore important that the next dose should be given half an hour before the effects of the previous dose wear off. But not everyone understands this, and if there is a delay and the PD becomes out of control people may think the dose is not strong enough <u>and increase the dosage</u> with the very worst results, which the sufferer is not fit at that moment to reject.

Professional carers are also under stress, and very busy and anxious to do the best for their residents. They are inclined therefore to try to simplify their medication routines, which is doubly upsetting to a PD sufferer. Firstly, because they may be anxious and distressed when they are no longer able to control their own medication, and then of course when any delay allows the PD to take over their bodies a bit more.

It should be emphasised again and again to all carers, both professional and amateur, that the timing and content of PD medication should never be altered without the doctor's or the home carer's consent. I do not know of any sufferer from PD who takes medication at regular, four hourly intervals and so I am afraid that in these establishments, Day Centres, Hospitals, Respite Care Homes etc, there ought to be a special timetable for the administration of each individual Parkinsonian's drugs. This can be one of the most comforting aspects of a stay with them; and the staff also needs to understand that the stress of strange surroundings, and parting from familiar faces, can also cause the swallow to become more inadequate so that taking pills can be more difficult.

I know of two cases where lack of training, or was it a lack of sympathy, caused distress and misunderstanding all round. In the first a PD sufferer had to be hospitalised at short notice and his swallow almost packed up. The staff misunderstood this and reported the sick man as difficult and refusing medication'. 'He just held the pills in his mouth and then let them dribble out again'. What actually happened, of course, was that he could not make that final movement that would send the pills down his throat.

In the second case a very busy nurse hurried into someone's house to give the sufferer a much needed enema. It was unusual for her to come in the afternoon and she had not before seen him when he was 'OFF'. The fluster and bustle caused him to become quite rigid and unable to move at all. The nurse spent some ten minutes trying to get the patient out of his chair, urging him to 'come on, do', to co-operate and not to be so awkward. But nothing unlocked his limbs. Eventually she left, after writing in his report book 'Refused enema'. Blaming the poor man, already in pain and distress and desperately needing the enema, instead of realising that she had misunderstood the situation, her report might cause a less helpful approach from the next nurse who was sent to help him.

I will not write more about treatment and medication; but surely the lesson to be learned from this story, and from any others I could tell, is simply listen to the carer.

A FEW MISUNDERSTANDINGS

Professionals may find amateurs annoying but sometimes I do find the attitude of medical people to PD hard to understand. They seem unable to get away from the books and to use <u>their own</u> vast knowledge, kindness and anxiety to help.

For instance, I have heard of the following cases:-

A sufferer for thirteen years was suddenly told that she had not got PD only a benign tremor. She was taken off her drugs, all her drugs, which had controlled her shake (shake rather than tremor), and as a result became unable to anything for herself at all.

Her shake became a wild, fast flying flap, and this flap increased under stress or when she tried to do anything. She could not feed herself, wash herself, walk, anything. We managed to get her an appointment with a specialist. She was quite at ease with him but found it distressing when he appeared to be assessing her <u>mental</u> capability by asking her the day of the week and the date. If you can only sit, flapping, in a chair with the television on continually to help to pass the time, the days of the week lose their importance. In fact at this moment I am not quite sure myself, without thinking about it, whether it is Tuesday or Wednesday, and I certainly do not know the date. She could not hold a newspaper nor go to the Day Centre nor bring in the milk. So of what importance was it whether it was Monday or Tuesday? Her husband cared for her devotedly, they had no visitors, every day was the same - one long flap. Poor lady, she was very worried that he thought she was becoming insane. Perhaps he could have been a little more tactful in his investigations?

Another test involved identifying the smell coming from three bottles. Perhaps this was necessary to check the sense of smell or the ability of recall, but the patient again was worried as she did not recognise one scent. She was not a cook and she may never have known the smell of vanilla. But her inability to recognise it had her really wound up and worried. What would that mean? Had she got something else wrong with her as well? Did PD do something to your nose?

Some patients find their check up worrying; they resent the shortness of their appointment. Some do not like the things they are asked to do, such as writing down a nursery rhyme. There may be some significance in this that escapes us, but I think elderly dignified men with a high IQ would rather write down something more in keeping with their lifestyle.

A sufferer living alone had his medication changed at his half yearly appointment with a consultant. 'Let me know how you get on with this' he was told. A few days later a neighbour reported that he was in a very poor way (and of course that being so he was not <u>able</u> to let anyone know). The doctor was called and referred him back to his consultant - who sent him another appointment for <u>six months ahead</u>! A private appointment had therefore to be arranged for him, with a promise of funding if possible. But he died from other causes very shortly afterwards. It was lucky that he had such good neighbours that they were able to call the doctor when they saw the change.

DO OUTSIDERS REALLY UNDERSTAND PD
AND TREAT THE SUFFERER AND CARER WITH KINDNESS?

Of course we all know the kind and healthy people who shout at all sick people as if they were deaf. They are doing their best, I expect, but it would help if they took trouble to learn a little more about the problems and forgot their own embarrassment in their wish to help others.

We also probably have met the elderly type who regards any illness that isn't actually a person covered with spots or a man with no legs as 'malade imaginaire', making a fuss, putting it on, which 'isn't done'. Why he should regard his ex-comrades as suddenly becoming whingers I do not know, unless it makes him feel safe from developing the same problems as they have. And of course it also gives him a standing as someone who would never complain about any bodily failing or incapacity himself, and saves him from having to offer to help the poor carer. But of course when he develops something himself it will be quite different and not at all *imaginaire.*

I hope that by the time you have finished reading this (only a few more pages!) you will understand some of the problems of PD and act accordingly. I know that I am not a professional with professional training but, after all, professional training is usually the result of learning from the experience of others. A condition like PD must be studied when the person is at ease, and when the visitor has plenty of time and is known and respected, NOT in the artificial, unnatural, stressful conditions of a clinic or hospital. There you see only a segment of the whole problem. There is not time to ask all the questions, and there certainly is not time to listen to the halting, slow reply, nor do you see the sufferer and carer under normal conditions and in their own home, with their children's photographs about - and even, perhaps, photos of them, themselves, in their younger days, from which you can learn a lot.

I would ask outsiders to respect at every stage the dignity of the sufferer and the family. It is not nice to find your parent has become a silent, shuffling, drooling old person in clothes that are now too big for their shrunken frame. But the parent is still their parent, and the soul and spirit is still inside the changed body, and their feelings of love and respect make the pain the greater. It is only the body language, the language you read from the body, which is now distorted. It would be easier to understand and accept if the person was in a wheelchair, and certainly easier to explain to the neighbours. But, alas, many PD sufferers fight against accepting the wheelchair and they still try to reach the loo instead of using a bottle; in both cases often with a disastrous result.

THOUGHTLESS OR UNINTENTIONAL KINDNESS

If someone is in scruffy clothes with a hangdog expression one is inclined to take a rather patronising attitude unlike one's attitude to an upright, well dressed, well shaved person with a loud voice and an air of command. It is the natural instinct of the herd to push the weakling out.

Sometimes I have noticed this reaction to people who are unsteady on their pins, with wispy hair, uncertain where they are going. Or if they are just crouched down quiet and sad in their chair while the others do the talking. You, too, may have heard this sort of thing:-

'Come on now; take your pills properly this time. Don't hold them in your mouth, <u>swallow</u> them, <u>swallow them</u> Mr .....' (or worse still using the Christian name);
'I can't wait here all day, hurry up, do';
'Put your jacket on yourself then - but you'll be late...';
'Hold your head up. How can I put your food in if you sit like that?'.

And I have even seen an attendant feed a sufferer while turned away talking to a friend.

'You go on' (to a fellow attendant) 'I'll bring Jack when he has been to the toilet' (or 'I've toiletted Jack'). 'We don't want any more trouble do we, Jack?';
'I can't understand if you speak so fast. Speak slowly. All right, write it down then - oh no, of course she can't write either, can she?'.

I have also heard this sort of ignorant criticism:-

'She leads him a dance';
'He is doing it on purpose to make it more difficult for her';
'He is just being naughty' (Naughty! How can anyone so speak of a person suffering from PD. That word, so often used by the ignorant, makes my blood boil).
'She promised she would never put him in a home, but he is completely unhelpful and she will have to do so soon' (this in the sufferer's hearing);
'He could manage perfectly well if he wanted to';
'Just like his mother - spoilt and bone idle'.

This sort of critical, unkind, arrogant and bossy attitude may be passed down, as I have said already, by trained outsider carers to their new assistants. The assistants may even copy them, thinking they are learning their craft. But please <u>do as you would be done by</u>. If you develop PD later you may be cared for by those who are training now, so please be a good ambassador for PD, explaining and training. Do not accept that PD people need a firm hand or an unsympathetic attitude. <u>It simply is not true</u>. They need patience, friendship and support. Hurrying and harassment only makes them worse and the Outsider's job that much harder.

THE HOME CARER, OR INSIDER
- HOW YOU CAN HELP THEM

The carer is probably the partner of some years' standing - or, as I have found a number of times lately, it may be a happy well-balanced second marriage after the death of the original partners. In either case the couple were looking forward to years of easy companionship, especially as they are very often of pensionable age.

They may have discussed old age and agreed that they would care for each other at home and would never put their partner 'away'.

There may be other health problems, as is bound to happen as we get older, rheumatism, angina, digestive problems, forgetfulness. Because PD does not have immediately recognisable outward signs, the PD person may be considered the healthier of the two and it should be he who should ease the burden of the other.

-oOo-

Please protect the couple, therefore, from the criticism of neighbours and even their own family, who think that they have a right to judge them and to tell them what they should be doing, and even how they ought to be 'managing' the Parkinsonism.

Give a real boost to the couple's morale by showing them how much you admire the good job they are doing, caring for each other, and make sure the family and friends you know admire them. Help them to come to terms with the word 'disabled' - it can be a very big step to realise that they are now in that category - and be ready with information on all the aids and support available.

If either becomes incontinent arrange for advice to be available. My age group still feels it is not quite nice to talk about such things, and shaming that we could be like that. But without help incontinence can take over and almost destroy people's social lives. Make sure they realise that it is not shaming but a natural sequence of living so long - or even possibly an infection that if reported to the doctor can be cleared up quite simply. Stress will make it worse, so when people say 'he wet himself on purpose' they only show up their ignorance and that they still do not understand the problem of STRESS. When talking to a carer try and mention incontinence quietly and naturally as something normal and easily helped and they may then find it possible to ask for help.

It is an 'open secret' among professionals that tea, coffee etc, can encourage incontinence, but I have never heard it mentioned in talks on PD, where stiffness of limbs can delay the arrival at the loo. Perhaps it would be kind to bring this to the notice of carers? However, elderly people may never have had much to do with doctors, health centres, and the other services and they do not understand the language or what the various initials stand for. Please explain everything to them in simple English. It is rather unkind to use technical jargon to someone you are meant to help. You may be the only link to all that is available. And the jargon changes, too, so that they may be out of date.

An example of this is 'therapy'. A word in daily use among professionals. It is tacked onto three very separate ways of helping people. But if someone has just been diagnosed as having PD (and this is a terrible shock to the family and they may need a lot of support) it will be something they have not heard before and will not understand, especially if elderly and rather deaf. Speech Therapist, Occupational Therapist, Physiotherapist - what does it all mean?

I very often get calls from members of the family, or even the next of kin, asking for an explanation of PD - nobody has told them anything etc, etc. The younger members of a family will be the ones who will support and help their parents and they should be given as much time and counselling as possible - or told of the existence of those who can. So often there is an expression of relief when they have talked over the problems and health problems and they are then able to give the carer the understanding help he or she needs; if the family understands PD they can come to terms with it, and plan how best to cope with it in the years to come.

'Managing' PD with medication is very important, but the quality of family life and emotional support is equally so. A slowly developing, insidious, possibly unattractive and not easily understood condition does not attract the same sympathy that the illnesses and tragedies of young people may receive. Nor is it 'newsworthy'.

Neighbours will still be annoyed if the house and garden are not kept up to standard. It can lower the tone of the neighbourhood. Maybe one of the youth organisations, St John Cadets, Guides, Scouts, Boys Brigade etc, could be encouraged to 'adopt' the garden. They might pass a badge doing it, and they would certainly learn about 'caring' and might well become friends with the owners of the garden. It might also, of course, draw a PD person out of his shell to see young people working among his flowers.

One can often recognise a Parkinsonian garden; it has nice things growing in it, but the grass has become uncontrolled, the weeds have enjoyed a season in the flower beds and the paint may need touching up on the gate and window sills. Cats may have done their worst. Like its owner the garden has gradually lost its pristine appearance and needs support and help. With PD there may be no obvious sign, like a white stick or a crutch, to show the neighbours that there is now something wrong; nothing for outsiders to recognise and so elicit understanding. In fact the outward signs of PD can be very similar to alcohol abuse. Not good for the neighbourhood.

Remember, also, that PD sufferers may have slow reactions. They may take a long time to respond to a cheery wave or "Morning", by which time the speaker will have turned the corner and be out of earshot. This can antagonise people. "Always was a difficult woman... Now she doesn't even answer. My wife believes she's taken to the bottle... Shouldn't be surprised. Their garden is a disgrace. And her husband looks exhausted. 'Spect she leads him a dance. What a life for a man".

But do the neighbours do anything to help or do they 'keep themselves to themselves'?

GETTING OUT AND ABOUT

Beyond the difficulty of finding transport and the difficulty of getting in and out of a car, there are many reasons why people may not want to go out, or appear not to welcome an invitation to do so. I have heard it said that 'only those who bother to come to our meetings are really interested in the Branch and really members of the Parkinson's Disease Society'. I can understand this point but I disagree with it totally. People usually approach a Society which offers to help them with problems either when they are newly diagnosed, or when they feel isolated and need information or help. They may well be housebound and need the feeling of support that membership of an organisation for sufferers and carers like themselves can give.

Then why do some people not want to come to meetings or Day Centres and meet other people? I have listed some of the reasons below. If an invitation is refused or not taken up I think we should try to find out tactfully why not, in case we can help in other ways.

They may no longer have the means of transport and do not wish to use a taxi, especially in the evenings;

Their partner may suffer from nausea, or be incontinent or suffer from agoraphobia or claustrophobia (all possible effects of PD or of their medication);

The sufferer's clothes may be stained or ill-fitting and they don't want to be seen, or to see others who may be worse than they are - a sign of things to come?;

They may be loners; they may never have been good mixers. (NB: Were they always like this or was this a sign of incipient PD?);

They may suffer from deafness which causes distress in crowds;

Some doctors are known to advise newly diagnosed sufferers not to attend PD meetings as they could find it depressing;

The journey to meetings may be too far, in another town maybe where they 'will know nobody';

They may not have established a rapport with the visitor from a branch who first invited them to come to a meeting;

The meetings may be after dark when they do not like to be out; or at the sufferer's OFF times, or at a time when their family comes to see them;

They may not have understood that the meetings are free;

They may think of it as charity, and they don't like that;

The sufferer may not like to eat in public because of his shake;

The loos may be difficult, the building may be too hot or too cold, the entrance may be difficult - or maybe the carer may simply fear that these difficulties will arise;

People may not like to explain that they do not want to accept an invitation because the transport offered is not suitable. I know of a well meaning man who raised a great deal of money to buy a small coach for disabled people in his village, and painted on its side 'The Village of .....'s Gift to the Disabled'. Then he was hurt that no-one wanted to be seen inside it!

They wanted time to think about the invitation perhaps because it clashed with their favourite TV programme;

They wanted to forget about the PD and were worried they would hear unpalatable truths;

They may not like the sort of meeting offered or may not feel at ease with the other people attending. PD strikes every level of intelligence and upbringing and you cannot please everyone.

In charitable organisations there is sometimes a feeling that anything offered to someone should be accepted with cries of joy. But it may not be the sort of thing that people like doing or having or seeing. However, the first refusal (in a quiet PD voice) can brand that person as 'ungrateful' and they may keep that reputation forever. I do not want to over-emphasise this but I have seen it happen more than once. One man I know once refused a charitable load of logs at Christmas, collected, sawn up and delivered free round the town by an excellent organisation. It was a cold day and he just said that he did not want them, thank you, and shut the door. The kind hearted people felt hurt and snubbed and he was struck off their list. It was some time before they found out what had really happened; only a few days previously his son and daughter-in-law had given him a new electric fire and bricked up the old wood-burning fireplace. This was to make life easier for him, now his wife had died. But he was deeply hurt by this, because their open fire had always been something his wife and he had enjoyed and when the load of logs came round it was like salt in the wound. If only the log people had realised what had happened it might have comforted him to have a received a basket of Christmas fare or something that did not remind him of the past.

They were just too tired.

FOR THE CARER,
SOME THINGS THAT MAY HELP

These are all simple things, but they are tips that have been passed on to me by carers and sufferers, so I gladly pass them on to you.

1.   That Old Black Magic: When a sufferer gets 'stuck to the floor' put something black on the floor in front of their feet and for some reason this will often enable them to step off (and over) the blackness and continue walking. You may have to keep placing it in front of them on a bad day. No-one knows why this works - hence the name I have given it.

2.   A Rolling Pin: This needs watching and should not be left on the floor but it is useful to encourage a person to keep their legs in better condition. Give it to them when they are sitting for some time. If they place their feet on the pin and roll it backwards and forwards it will encourage a good supply of blood to the feet. It is very tiring to do (makes your knees ache) so do not expect them to continue for long. Little and often is the answer. It is a good idea to use it just before someone is going to stand up. It may also help those sufferers who get very cold knees and thighs. <u>Remember to pick it up before the sufferer gets to his feet</u>...

3.   Foam lagging for water pipes can be bought very cheaply by the metre. Cut a short piece off and use it to bind round hand utensils, knife, fork, pen, paintbrush etc, to make them fatter and therefore easier to grip. In fact the user is more likely then to work from their elbow instead of the wrist or fingers and this is good because the movements will be more positive. The writing is more legible and bolder and the food is more easily conveyed to the mouth. Foam handles can be made more cheaply than the special utensils found in the shops which are sometimes awkward and slippery to hold.

4.   Speech, Exercise and Relaxation tapes can be bought from the Parkinson's Disease Society, but they are expensive. Perhaps a Day Centre or other group could share them?

5.   The Parkinson's Disease Society produces some booklets which have helpful information. But, once more, the effects of PD are so varied that it is difficult to give good advice to all, without painting a gloomy picture. The secondary effect of this is that cheery next of kin reading some of the booklets may not realise what a strain caring for a sufferer can be and their attitude may contain some exasperation in it, which does not help anyone. Carers need to be admired and also supported and helped, not told they are making too much of it all. Let there be no mistake. To be told that you, or your partner, have PD is bad enough. The problems and the exhaustion and the loss of the person they married is bad enough. If the nearest and dearest then misunderstand, or even poo-poo the depth of the difficulties and think that you are exaggerating then things get even blacker. Sufferers and carers need all the help and understanding they can get. They do not want to be told they are making an unnecessary fuss.

6.   A chair that helps people get in and out of it. This can be supplied through the statutory services. It is one of the most inhibiting procedures for a sufferer, and extremely bad for the carer's back, to have to be hoisted up at a difficult angle. But if sufferers can get out of a chair when they want to, on their own, they regain a lot of their freedom, for it is <u>comparatively</u> easy to walk about. Being able to change your position or stand for a few minutes can also help to prevent pressure sores.

Do not be like one OT who told me that he would not provide a chair for a gentleman <u>yet</u>, because he might <u>become reliant</u> on it... I still cannot work out his reasons for this. Sadly the couple had to go to a home because without the chair the PD sufferer could not get in and out of his chair and provide meals for his arthritic wife.

7.   A Spoon: Any old spoon which can be bent at right angles may make it easier for a sufferer to get it to his mouth.

8.   Ordinary wooden clothes pegs can be clipped on to pages, newspaper sheets or any other fiddly items to make them easier to grasp.

9.   An iced drink immediately before a meal stimulates the swallow and may enable a sufferer to eat more quickly. It has been suggested to me that a cloth wrung out in very cold water and placed on the jaw line might also stimulate the swallow, but I have not heard of anyone who did this. The Speech Therapist should be able to help overcome the problem of the swallow.

10.   Nylon sheets or clothes may help sufferers to turn in bed.

11.   Labelled boxes, jam jars, tins etc, so that the day's medicines can be counted out all at one time. People may forget if they have taken their 11.30 dose but a glance at the boxes will show if '11.30' is still there. People must remember to keep them out of the reach of children, but the children could be asked to decorate the jars/boxes with pictures or large letters. It is also possible to buy pill boxes for a day's supply, but they are inclined to be fiddly and difficult for PD hands to open and get the pills out.

12.   Chewing gum (I believe Excel is very good) will help to control dribbling and encourage swallowing in the less badly affected. But I am told that chewing gum can have a bad effect on some dentures, so the dentist should be contacted first.

13.   A two-handed oven cloth can be laid over the arm of a chair and used for a supply of tissues. The unused ones go in the outer 'hand' and the less attractive go in the 'hand' next to the sufferer's body, out of sight.

14.   Plates that can keep the food hot and palatable for longer if the sufferer has difficulty in swallowing. Other suggestions are:-

   (a) Put the food into a small bowl rather than a soup plate so that the spoon/fork can be dragged up the side more easily; possibly it is easier to keep food hot in such a container?

   (b) Only serve a small portion of the food at a time, while the rest keeps warm on the stove. It is less discouraging to a sufferer to clear the plate, then to have a little more, than to feel they will never finish it all ...

15.   A board under the mattress, where shoulders to hips will be, can give a person a grab hold to help to turn. It should only stick out a few inches from the bed and be padded. Alternatively, tie a rope right round the bed frame and make it loose enough for the sufferer to grab.

   I am told that it is often the inability to move about in bed that causes his body to wake him up during the night, and it is only then that they feel they should get up and go to the loo. We do not realise how much we move about in bed at night (thus preventing pressure sores). If someone's body becomes PD stiff then the body will wake the brain. Use anything that makes it easier for the sufferer to move more easily and it may well be that they will not then have a such a distressing sleep pattern.

16. Getting in and out of a car presents many difficulties and the thought of having to do so may cause the sufferer to stiffen up. I give a few well tried hints, but they must be adapted to the person's needs:-

(a) Park the car well away from the kerb.

(b) Ask the sufferer for their blue card.

(c) If in a busy area put the boot up, and leave the wheelchair or zimmer where other drivers can see it.

(d) Place a plastic bag on the seat and a small soft cushion on top (this will enable the passenger to be swung round once sitting down).

(e) Relax the passenger by saying there is lots of time.

(f) A piece of material some 30-40cm (12-15") deep and 122cm (48") + long can be placed under the passenger's armpits, dropping down to her hips. If you hold the ends and lean back slightly to keep the material taut you will give the passenger a great feeling of security and they will be able to manoeuvre themselves into the car without fearing they are going to fall, and their hands will be free. Leave the material in place for getting out again.

(g) Remember the danger of hitting their heads on the top of the door space.

(h) Wait a second before you try to slide the passenger round on the cushion, bringing in the legs. And then do up the safety belt.

(i) Do not talk all the time when a passenger is getting into the car. They want to concentrate.

17. If possible have a list of disabled loos with you and know which ones are always open and easily accessible.

18. Old telephone directories can be used in many places where something needs to be raised. For instance the bottom of the bed (put the directories under the feet of the bed), or chairs. If a person's body is tipped slightly back and the TV raised a little above the level of their heads their bodies will be at a better angle, their chests expanded and they may breathe more deeply and thus improve the supply of oxygen to their brains. They can also be used to raise the table legs so that a wheelchair can be pushed right up to the table.

19. Finally, remember that the charitable caring organisations, the Red Cross and St John Ambulance, hold stocks of 'comforts' to ease the life of sick people. Sometimes you will be asked to pay for the hire. All members of these organisations are trained in home nursing as well as first aid and are volunteers who can be asked to help in the home. They like to be asked, or all their training is wasted. They may also be available for 'sitting' with a person who cannot be left on their own. The ideal of St John Ambulance is to care for 'Our Masters the Sick'. Look these organisations up in the telephone directory (Red Cross will probably be under B for British, but St John will be under St John).

20. Talking Books, Talking Newspapers, Domiciliary visits from the Library Service all help to improve the quality of life of a PD family. And there are still quite a few travelling shops if you can find them. They should be registered with your local council.

These are all 'tricks' that I have been told over the years; of course none of them are as useful as a visit from the statutory services coming to advise you, but this may tide you over until they come. I think it is up to you to ask the Health Visitor at your Surgery to ask them to call.

IF YOU REALLY WANT TO HELP A PARKINSONIAN FAMILY

AVOID

changing the drug regime;

putting the sufferer into the wrong sort of ward, e.g. psychiatric. This can frighten both the sufferer and the carer, and make them think that perhaps there is a mental problem. And they are emotionally distressed too. To be in a ward with those who are unfortunately afflicted does not improve the quality of life of the Parkinsonian nor will it, therefore, give a true reading of their condition. Stress will build up very quickly. (On the other hand, if a sufferer is in a nice friendly ward they may well unwind and talk more than they have for years to fellow inmates);

trying to teach the sufferer to help himself more. Putting things too far away so that they have to stretch, telling them to go to the loo on their own when they are already disorientated and unsteady. This cannot be good nursing and can cause a lot of extra work for the staff;

forgetting to turn the sufferer every two hours if they are unable to turn themselves. If they have come in without pressure sores, they should go out the same way;

talking at them rather than to them;

using their Christian name without permission (especially if you are about 18 and they are 70+);

bossing; and especially avoid bossing in a loud voice so that the whole ward hears;

destroying their dignity;

forgetting they will probably suffer from constipation (very common in PD);

taking away their medication if they normally manage it themselves. If you are then unavoidably late in giving it to them they may quickly deteriorate and be unable to attract your attention. This is horrible for them and they will lose faith in you;

forgetting to tell the carer when they can see the doctor or consultant on his ward round (and do make sure they have transport);

thinking you can change the sufferer's behaviour, permanently. You can't;

expecting them to wear any old clothes. Make sure they wear their own. Remember the carer may have brought new ones to be worn in hospital;

hurrying sufferers when eating; Do give them a very cold drink first in the hope that this will activate their swallow. They may need help - avoid making them feel embarrassed. Would they be better on their own, or just with you?;

waking up a sufferer just because they are asleep 'at the wrong time'.

REMEMBER

that some drugs have to be taken within a certain time of taking food, so make sure there are no delays;

that some highly spiced foods, curry etc, will cause an odd reaction from the medication. Keep a list of any food that upsets the sufferer who may not be able to tell you himself.

WHEN YOU ARE CARING FOR A PARKINSONIAN

AVOID

trying to stimulate sufferers all day long (their day is tiring enough already);

trying to teach or re-teach them to do things that their PD bodies can no longer do, e g buttons, zips etc. You may achieve something for a short time but it will not be permanent;

leaving Parkinsonians sitting in one position for too long;

giving them chairs which encourage a slouching posture. Make sure that they have to look UP to the TV, preferable resting their heads slightly backwards;

putting a cushion behind their backs to help them sit up - it won't. Put the cushions under their armpits to give them some support;

judging their behaviour against the behaviour of anyone else you know who has PD - they are bound to be different;

sitting Parkinsonians together;

thinking that someone is asleep and need not be helped; possibly their back has given way and they have flopped onto the table;

thinking that a person is not interested, or is not going to answer, just because they take some time to reply.

REMEMBER

that the sufferer is at your Day Centre to <u>give their carer a rest</u>. Therefore it is important to send the sufferer home relaxed and not tired, fussed or over stimulated. As I said above it is unlikely that anything you teach the sufferer can be retained permanently because of the PD, so there is no point in insisting that they 'learn' how to do this or that;

a sufferer may become disorientated and try to go home. This is not 'running away' nor is it 'naughty'. In fact NEVER, EVER use the word 'naughty' in connection with a sufferer from PD;

if a carer or sufferer is not happy with your Day Centre or Hospital the carer may stop them coming. If they are happy it is a wonderful life save for the carer and a feather in your cap;

that journeys in cars or other transport should be as short as possible, for PD people may suffer from nausea. They are often incontinent and distressed by speed, bustle, moving sights outside the window, or even noise within the transport.

REMEMBER EVERYONE

PD medication often takes some time to act, with a bizarre result at first. To avoid this sufferers try to take their next medication before they have 'burnt up' the last lot. Trust their carer to ell you when they must have their next medication and stick rigidly to this and ensure that your staff do too;

to help sufferers to unscrew their bottles and provide drinks for them in good time. As the medication wears off the sufferer's condition may worsen and they will not be able to say or do things they normally can.

PLEASE DO NOT BE CROSS

or insulted or irritated if the carer has asked for the sufferer to be allowed to take their own medication at times different from the ward/day centre round. This is because they have learnt how to provide the best possible medication over the years. It is not for us to take offence or try to change their medication regime.

I am stressing this point because I have heard of a case only today where a sufferer was 'allowed' to control his own medication only after much argument. The medicine was then locked into a cupboard by his bed. When his condition worsened unexpectedly (which it can often do under stress or in strange surroundings) he was not able to put the key in the lock but on asking the nurse for help he was told to get on with it himself - he was in charge, wasn't he? No help was forthcoming. Was this tender loving care?

WORDS THAT CAN CONFUSE THE LAYMAN
(in alphabetical order)

CLIENT	this was used to denote the person needing help, but I think it has now been replaced by Service User. The statutory services are Service Providers I think. It does not mean that any money changes hands.
COMPLAIN	the doctor may say that a patient 'complains of ...' This only means that that is what someone has come to see him about.
FORMAL	The professionals are the FORMAL CARERS. Those looking after a partner at home are INFORMAL CARERS!
MANAGING	doctors 'manage' the care of the sufferer by prescribing his medicine.
SOCIAL	means, I think, the care of people in need outside the medical world.
SOCIAL WORKER	is therefore the person to whose care a person in need is allotted and who should be able to be contacted when things go wrong. They work very hard.
SPECIALTY	this is a word meaning the special department and interest of a Consultant. (Different spelling from speciality).
STATUTORY WORKER	is I think anyone employed by the Government to help people other than the medical profession themselves.
THERAPISTS	are people who try to improve things. They are trained professionals in a special branch of 'improving'. Speech Therapists try to help you improve your speech, breathing, swallow etc. Physiotherapists try to improve all your body's physical movements etc, and Occupational Therapists try to improve the arrangements in your home, especially after an accident, or when you are returning to your home after a stay in hospital. (That is very simplified). The point to remember is that there are three different types of therapist.

NB: I think the way some of these words are used causes confusion to elderly people. I am sorry that there is not room to quote some amusing examples of misunderstanding.

THANK YOU AND GOODBYE

I am grateful to you for reading as far as this; it shows that you really do care about people who suffer from PD and I hope that these notes have been of some help to you and enabled you to have a better, more gentle approach and appreciation of PD sufferers and their hardworking carers. PD really can tear a family apart.

I would like to thank all those friends who have talked to me about their problems and given me the examples I have quoted. I have tried in each case to prevent their being recognised.

There are so many more cases I would like to quote, and possibly should quote, but time and finance cannot permit at present. I will wait and see how this booklet is received.

I hope I have not appeared critical or disparaging of the care that is given by dedicated, wise and understanding caring staff. But there are many people who do not understand, who cannot put themselves in the sufferer's and carer's place. My wish has been to show them, probably the kindest people (and if so they will not mind my doing so), why it is necessary that they adjust their approach to Parkinsonians. And also to show all people what they can do to lessen the burden of these ravaged lives. As in so much it is necessary for them to go far beyond the halfway mark in helping people who can no longer help themselves.

My message throughout has been "do not believe for one moment that a Parkinsonian is trying to be difficult. He is battling against his PD as best he can". Keep quiet, show patience, do not push and hurry him with phrases such as 'you can if you want to', 'you did it all right yesterday'. Above all, perhaps, treat him with dignity.

And to all Parkinson's families I would say 'The more you show yourselves, the more you describe your problems to those formal carers, the more you ask for what you feel is what you need, or which would help you, then the more will be done for you and other PD families. Do not forget it is only you, the Insiders, who can really tell us, the Outsiders, what it is like and what you need. We are trying to help you - but are we doing the right thing? Only you can tell us.

Included at the back of this booklet are a few pages which may be of interest and a 'Hospital Sheet' which if completed might be of use when a sufferer had to go into hospital or had to have an operation. The sheet should be kept up to date and regarded as a sort of Parkinson's Passport to good care.

This book is dedicated to all carers and their sufferers, and to those of my friends who work so hard to help them. Any proceeds will go to a special fund recently set up by three friends for the welfare of suffers and their families. This fund has no administrative or office expenses; every penny raised goes direct to help people with PD.

Pam McClintock
Wareham
Dorset
BH20 4PR

JIM

He was always an awkward chap. Never speaking to anyone, never looking at anyone, never a smile. Just plain difficult. It wasn't our fault that he had Parkinson's, and yet he took it out on us all. So demanding. So difficult.

Take yesterday for instance. You know what it is like here around lunchtime, everyone wanting to go to the loo, having to be got ready. Kitchen going spare. So I thought I'd get to old Jim a bit early and about 12 I popped my head round the door. "Hullo, Jim" I said, nice as pie, "lunch in half an hour. Do you want to use the toilet?"

Never an answer, never a smile. Didn't even both to turn his head. "All right" I said, "don't worry" and went on to Mrs K.

Came half past we started to serve the lunches and I took Jim's up to him. It was a nice lunch and I told him so. "Your favourite, Jim" I said, "Stew and mashed potatoes". I drew his table up and settled the tray down in front of him. All nice and hot and smelling really tasty.

So what do you think Jim said? Thank you? Oh no. Just when I had got everything ready for him and was leaving the room His Majesty spoke. "I want to go to the toilet" he said.

Well, it was enough to make an angel scream. Why couldn't he have told me before, or when I came in at 12? Why did he wait till I had fixed everything up ready for him to eat it? So I had to start again. Remove the table, get him out of the chair and take him along, and he making himself stiff and awkward as he could. And then we only just got there in time. Why couldn't he have been co-operative just once? Why couldn't he have said yes when I popped my head in at 12? No wonder the other girls call him names at times.

A MESSAGE FROM A SUFFERER
WHICH SHE DICTATED TO HELP YOU IN YOUR CARING

Parkinson's attacks the motor nerves and thus one's limbs and muscles do not always do what you expect them to do. You are also subject to involuntary jerking. I have punched and kicked whoever is on my left hand side more than once. Should either your neighbour or you yourself be eating or drinking at this time, the poor unsuspecting soul would possibly get their meal all over them. Embarrassing to say the least!

When a tremor affects your arms - these describing ever faster and bigger circles - you quite literally cannot control the limb nor yet let go of whatever you are holding. It is quite amazing how far a cup of tea will go! Your feet also 'freeze' to the ground and you CANNOT MOVE. Some well meaning person will say "Move over a bit will you, dear?" Move over! Don't you wish you could!

May I here speak a few words to all those dedicated people without whom we PD sufferers would never survive.

PLEASE NEVER WALK BACKWARDS IN FRONT OF US HOLDING OUR HANDS as this causes us to take little steps, and a longish stride is necessary to obtain balanced movement. The results of this 'backward shuffle' can be quite spectacular.

PLEASE DON'T KEEP US STANDING as we tend to fold up - not always gracefully - on the floor! Tell us all the news, and once you have stood up, manners compelling us to try to do the same, PLEASE GO!

PLEASE ALSO REMEMBER that we cannot wriggle around to get comfortable, so ensure we are comfortable before you leave us for the night.

I personally find getting in and out of cars very difficult. Our muscle response is slow and being told to 'swing your legs over' is like being told 'Just run up Everest, will you?'

TURNING is also nerve wracking; here the rules have to be strict. Remember, our feet often stick to the ground and will not unstick to order, so please BE VERY CAREFUL to see we are really mobile. Don't let us turn to close the door once we are out of the vehicle as, doing this, we are highly likely to fall flat on our faces. Not a pretty sight.

DRESSING AND UNDRESSING is also a sight to see and, on a bad day, rivals prime-time TV. The contortions one can get into have to be seen to be believed, many a time I have given up and spent the day in my nightdress and dressing gown.

Knickers and stockings present the biggest problem and often I have been over an hour trying to attach them to my person. A bit of assistance is really needed but not always available. I have lost all pride and sometimes feel that half the female population of my town have a nodding acquaintance with my underwear!

Try to have as much as possible opening down the front, putting up one's arms to try to insert them into sleeves is fraught with danger. I once tried this manoeuvre while alone in the flat and fell over backwards pulling a rack full of clothes on top of me. I was wedged tight between my bed and the wall, quite unable to move and suffocating under the clothes. Very scary!

ANOTHER HAZARD CONNECTED WITH DRESSING AND UNDRESSING is the loving helpful but not very skilful helper. I remember with mixed feelings the memorable night when two dear friends decided they would both help, unfortunately they were two individualists and could not co-ordinate their decisions. I was pulled all ways at once, with no strength to resist, with the result that I finally ended up with arms and head wedged into a tube of material and every prospect of remaining with my arms stuck up in the air!

WASHING ONESELF has a lot in common with dressing. The most useful gadget is a metal chair with the sloping seat called a 'perching stool' allowing one to draw up to the wash basin. Before I had this chair and while living alone, washing often had to be abandoned.

Eating is an occupation that is mirth-provoking or irritating, according to your viewpoint. You cannot cut anything up because you have no strength to apply the appropriate pressure. You cannot spear anything with a fork because you cannot co-ordinate two movements and to try to convey anything from plate to mouth by spoon....! Impossible.

If you are a helper at mealtimes it is a great kindness to remember small spoonfuls properly spaced. It is most upsetting to have your mouth full up and be unable to swallow it before the next lot arrives. Soups and all liquids are best dealt with by using a baby's drinking cup or straw I found.

Help is really essential, and it is a courtesy to draw as little attention to this degrading past-time as possible.

I hope these few anecdotes will help any Parkinsonians and their carers to see that, given the right attitude, it is still possible to have some kind of life. Learn to keep interested outside yourself and above all, keep your sense of humour. Laughter helps a lot. Laugh and the world laughs with you, weep and you weep alone.

I have to say that my life was saved by the Consultant who came to me after complaints of indifferent care given me by the previous Consultant. To him I had been an anonymous number on a list. To the older man I was a person with feelings and he treated me as such.

DOCTORS PLEASE NOTE: Patients are often highly intelligent, sensitive people and only too well aware of the lack of dignity that becomes their lot. Any consideration shown them is doubly appreciated. Remember also that if you see a patient in a clinic they are <u>well enough that day to get there</u>. But you only really know your patient's condition if you see them on a bad day in their own home. To widen YOUR understanding and knowledge jump at the chance of a Home Visit, and if you can arrange for that to be at the patient's bad time of day - so much the better.

EDITOR'S NOTE: The disabilities described here are one person's PD. Others have other difficulties. NO TWO CASES OF PD ARE THE SAME but always your understanding, your patience, your tolerance will ease the problems of the afflicted.